The DIY Guide to Methylene Blue

A Comprehensive Handbook for Safe and Efficient Use

Brent Andersen

1

Chapter One

DIY Guide to Methylene Blue

Methylene Blue: What Is It?

Methylene Blue, also known as methylthioninium chloride, is a synthetic dye with a variety of applications in medicine, biology, and chemistry. It appears as a dark green crystalline powder, which turns blue when dissolved in water. Chemically, it is a redox agent, capable of both donating and accepting electrons, making it valuable in various oxidative-reductive reactions.

Methylene blue is mostly used in medicine to treat methemoglobinemia, a disorder in

which the blood's supply of
methemoglobin reduces the
body's ability to release oxygen
into the tissues. Additionally, it is
used as a cyanide poisoning
antidote and is being investigated
as a potential cognitive enhancer
for neurodegenerative disorders
such as Alzheimer's. It contain
antifungal as well as antibacterial
qualities as well.

Methylene blue is used in
aquarium maintenance to treat
fish illnesses and stop fungal
infections in fish eggs, in addition
to its medical uses. It is an
essential staining agent in biology
that makes cells and tissues more

visible under a microscope. In many other laboratory chemical reactions, its function as a redox indicator is also important.

It's important to handle Methylene Blue safely. Nausea, lightheadedness, and infrequently, severe allergic reactions are possible adverse effects. It can interact with pharmaceuticals like antidepressants, causing serotonin syndrome, and is not recommended for people with diseases like glucose-6-phosphate dehydrogenase (G6PD) insufficiency.

Chapter Two

Why a Do-It-Yourself Guide?

A DIY Methylene Blue handbook has multiple significant uses:

1. Accessibility

Making a do-it-yourself guide increases accessibility to Methylene Blue knowledge for a wider range of people, including those without professional expertise in science or medicine. This enables people to use Methylene Blue for a variety of purposes in a safe and efficient manner.

2. Education

The handbook gives
comprehensive information about
Methylene Blue, including its
characteristics, applications, and
possible hazards. Users are
encouraged to utilize it
responsibly and intelligently,
which lowers the risk of misuse or
mishaps.

3. Practical Applications

A do-it-yourself manual provides
useful, detailed directions for
making and using Methylene
Blue. This covers sourcing,
measuring, mixing, and dosing—
all essential for reaching the
intended results, be they

scientific, medical, or
recreational.

4. Safety

Safety is the most important
factor to consider when working
with chemicals. The extensive
safety protocols, possible side
effects, contraindications, and
interaction warnings included in
the handbook guarantee that
users are well-informed about the
safe handling of Methylene Blue.

5. Cost-Effectiveness

Buying pre-made Methylene Blue
solutions might be costly for a
variety of uses. A do-it-yourself
guide enables people to make

their own solutions, which could result in cost savings and increase the viability of using Methylene Blue on a regular basis.

6. Flexibility

Applications for Methylene Blue are numerous and include biological staining, aquarium maintenance, and medical therapies. The usability and relevancy of a DIY guide are increased since it covers these many applications and offers specific instructions and advice for each.

7. Inventiveness and Trials

A do-it-yourself guide promotes creativity and experimentation among researchers and enthusiasts. It gives users the safety and knowledge base they need to investigate new Methylene Blue applications and usage in their respective fields.

A helpful resource that democratizes information, encourages safe procedures, and increases the adaptability and accessibility of this significant substance is a do-it-yourself Methylene Blue handbook.

Historical Applications and Findings

Methylene blue has a long and illustrious history that dates back to the 19th century, filled with important discoveries and uses.

Finding out

• **Synthesis:** German chemist Heinrich Caro created Methylene Blue for the first time in 1876 as a component of the dye industry.

• **First Medical usage:** The first medical usage of this substance dates back to 1891, when renowned scientist Paul Ehrlich found that it might be used to cure malaria.

Early Medical Application

• **Treatment for Malaria:**
Ehrlich's discovery made it
possible for the medicine to be
used against malaria, especially
in the early 20th century.

• **Antiseptic characteristics:**
Methylene Blue has been used to
treat a variety of wounds and
infections because to its
antiseptic characteristics.

Staining and Microscopy

• **Biological Staining:** This stain
has been used extensively in
histology and microbiology to aid
in the visualization of cells and
tissues under a microscope. It

works very well for recognizing cell architecture and staining germs.

Scientific Research

• **Redox Reactions:** Because of its qualities as a redox agent, it is useful in scientific research on the study of electron transport and cellular respiration.

• **Treatment for Methemoglobinemia:** During the middle of the 20th century, it was discovered that Methylene Blue was a useful remedy for methemoglobinemia, a disorder that results in an inefficient release of oxygen from hemoglobin to bodily tissues.

Second World War

- **Antimalarial Use:** Methylene Blue was used to treat malaria in soldiers during World War II, particularly in areas where the illness was common.

Modern Application

- **Neurodegenerative Research:** Because of its neuro-protective and cognitive-enhancing qualities, methylene blue has recently been the subject of research into its potential benefits in treating neurodegenerative disorders, including Parkinson's and Alzheimer's disease.

- **Antibacterial Properties:** Due to its antibacterial qualities, it is still utilized in a variety of medical and non-medical settings, such as urinary antiseptics and aquarium maintenance.

Chapter Three

Chemical Properties of Methylene Blue

A synthetic substance with unique chemical properties, methylene blue is necessary for a variety of applications.

Chemical Formula

• Formula.: C16H18ClN3S

• Structure: It is made composed of a sulfur atom, two methyl groups, and a phenothiazine ring system.

Physical Appearance

• Color: Powdery dark green crystals.

• Color of Solution: When dissolved in water, this substance yields a deep blue solution.

Solubility

• Solubility in Water: Very soluble in water.

• Solubility in Other Solvents: Alcohol slightly dissolves it.

The chemicals stability

• Stability: In typical circumstances, stable.

• Storage: To ensure stability, keep out of direct sunlight and moisture. Store in a cool, dry place.

Redox Properties

• Redox Activity: Participates in chemical reactions by acting as a redox agent and receiving and donating electrons.

• Electron Transfer: It is helpful in a variety of oxidative and reductive processes because it promotes electron transfer reactions.

Acid-Base Characteristics

• pKa: About 2.5 in water, meaning it has the ability to function as a weak acid.

• Ionization: When dissolved in water, it forms a stable chloride ion ($Cl-$).

Reactivity of Chemicals

• Types of Reactions: Takes part in electron transfer, complex formation, and oxidation-reduction reactions.

• Indicators: Changes color in response to oxidation state changes, serving as a redox indicator in chemical analysis.

Uses for Chemical Properties

• Medication: Used as an antidote for cyanide poisoning, to treat methemoglobinemia, and maybe for therapeutic purposes in neurology.

- Biology: Used in microscopy to improve the visibility of cell structures as a biological stain.

- Industry: Used as a redox indicator in analytical chemistry and as a textile dye in the past.

The structure and composition of methylene blue

Composition:

- Formula for Chemistry: $C_{16}H_{16}ClN_3S$

The molecular weight is roughly 319.85 g/mol.

Structure:

• Core Structure: Methylene Blue is a member of the phenothiazine chemical class.

• Basic Structure: It is made up of the following elements in a tricyclic phenothiazine ring system:

• Central Ring: Consists of one sulfur atom (S) and two nitrogen atoms (N).

• Substituents: The nitrogen atoms are joined to two methyl (CH3) groups.

• Chlorine atom (Cl) is connected to the aromatic ring.

Chemical Bonds:

• Aromatic Ring System: Conjugated aromatic rings are a part of Methylene Blue's structure and give it its distinctive color and electrical characteristics.

• Ionic Form: Methylene Blue usually exists as Methylene Blue chloride in aqueous solutions, which improves its solubility and stability.

Groups with Functions:

• Methyl groups (CH_3): These groups are linked to nitrogen atoms and affect their solubility and chemical reactivity.

• Chlorine Atom (Cl): A halogen substituent that modifies the stability and solubility of the compound as well as its physical and chemical characteristics.

Structure:

• Color: A dark green crystalline powder whose conjugated aromatic system gives rise to a blue tint in solution.

• Solubility: Due to its high water solubility, it can be used in a variety of watery applications in biology, chemistry, and medicine.

Chapter Four

Methylene Blue's Stability and Solubility

Solubility:

• Water Solubility: Methylene Blue has a high water solubility, which is useful for applications using aqueous solutions.

• Solubility in Other Solvents: Although it is mostly soluble in water, it is also marginally soluble in alcohol and other organic solvents.

Stability:

• Chemical Stability: When stored in a regular manner and maintained away from heat, light, and moisture, methylene blue is generally stable.

• Storage Requirements: To avoid deterioration and preserve its chemical integrity, store it in a cold, dry location.

• Light Sensitivity: It is light-sensitive, and extended exposure to light may cause alterations in its chemical composition or other deterioration.

Practical Consideration:

• Preparation: To guarantee optimal potency and stability, Methylene Blue solutions should be made freshly as needed.

• Usage: To preserve efficacy, solutions should be used promptly after preparation and kept in light-resistant containers.

• Handling: To avoid contamination and guarantee precise dosing, careful handling is necessary during preparation and storage.

Comprehending Methylene Blue's solubility and stability properties is essential for its efficient use in a variety of applications, such as biological staining, analytical chemistry, and medical therapies. For it to be effective and provide consistent results, handling and storage procedures must be followed correctly.

The way that Methylene Blue works

Methylene blue is useful in a wide range of biological, chemical, and medicinal applications because it works through multiple important mechanisms:

1. Redox Processes

• Electron Transfer: Methylene Blue functions as a redox agent in biological reactions, easily taking up and giving up electrons.

• Mitochondrial Function: Promotes oxidative phosphorylation and electron transport, two processes essential to the synthesis of cellular energy.

2. Methemoglobinemia Treatment

• Methemoglobin Conversion: Methylene Blue changes ferric iron (Fe^{3+}) in methemoglobin back to ferrous iron (Fe^{2+}), restoring hemoglobin's ability to carry oxygen efficiently in cases of methemoglobinemia.

3. Antioxidants Properties

• Free Radical Scavenging: Reduces oxidative stress and cellular damage by scavenging reactive oxygen species (ROS).

This process serves as an antioxidant.

4. Effects of Neuroprotection

• Mitochondrial Protection: May be helpful in neurodegenerative illnesses such as Parkinson's and Alzheimer's. It shields neurons from oxidative damage and maintains mitochondrial function.

5. Antimicrobial Intensity

• Antibacterial and Antifungal: Its ability to exhibit antimicrobial actions against specific bacteria and fungi makes it useful as a urinary antiseptic and in the treatment of infections.

6. Staining by Biochemistry

• Cellular staining: This stain is frequently used in biological and medical laboratories to improve the contrast and visibility of cells and tissues under a microscope, supporting research and diagnostic efforts.

7. Indicator Chemical

• Redox Indicator: Methylene Blue is used in titrations and other chemical investigations as a redox indicator in analytical chemistry. It changes color according to its oxidation state.

Safety Observations:

• Methylene Blue can cause adverse effects like nausea, vomiting, and in rare cases, severe allergic responses, even though it is generally thought to be safe when taken as indicated.

• Because it can cause hemolysis, it should be used carefully in people with certain conditions, such as glucose-6-phosphate dehydrogenase (G6PD) deficiency.

Chapter Five

Methylene Blue's Mode of Action in Biological Systems

Methylene blue is useful for a variety of applications in biology, medicine, and research because it affects biological systems through a number of important mechanisms:

1. Redox Properties

• Electron Transfer: In biochemical activities, methylene blue functions as a redox agent, accepting and donating electrons.

• Cellular respiration: Promotes the creation of cellular energy (ATP synthesis) by facilitating electron transport in mitochondria.

2. Methemoglobinemia Treatment

• Methemoglobin Conversion: In methemoglobinemia, ferric iron (Fe^{3+}) in methemoglobin is converted back to ferrous iron (Fe^{2+}) by Methylene Blue, regaining the protein's capacity to bind and transport oxygen.

3. Activity of Antioxidants

• Free Radical Scavenging: Reduces oxidative stress and shields cells from harm by scavenging reactive oxygen species (ROS). This process serves as an antioxidant.

4. Effects of Neuroprotection

• Mitochondrial Protection: May have significance for neurological illnesses such as Alzheimer's, and it shields neurons from oxidative damage and promotes mitochondrial function.

5. Antimicrobial Characteristics

• Antibacterial and Antifungal: Its ability to exhibit antimicrobial actions against specific bacteria and fungi makes it useful as a urinary antiseptic and in the treatment of infections.

6. Staining by Biochemistry

• Cellular staining: This stain is frequently used in biological and medical labs to improve the visibility of cell structures under a microscope, supporting research and diagnoses.

7. Chemical Indicator

• Redox Indicator: used in titrations and chemical studies, this tool changes color according to the oxidation state of the material to indicate redox reactions in analytical chemistry.

Chapter Six

Common Applications of Methylene Blue in Science and Medicine

A flexible substance, methylene blue has a number of well-established and developing uses in the scientific and medical domains.

Medicine:

1. Treatment of Methemoglobinemia:

• Mechanism: Converts methemoglobin (Fe^{3+}) back to hemoglobin (Fe^{2+}), restoring oxygen-carrying ability in blood.

• Clinical Use: Treating congenital and acquired methemoglobinemia in an emergency.

2. Antidote cyanide poisoning:

• Mechanism: Aids in detoxification by converting cyanide to less poisonous cyanate, which facilitates cellular respiration.

• Clinical Use: Especially in acute situations, utilized as a component of cyanide poisoning therapy protocols.

3. Urinary Antiseptic:

• Mechanism: Used to treat urinary tract infections, it

demonstrates antibacterial activity against bacteria.

• Clinical Use: As a support treatment for urinary tract infections, especially in cases where other measures are not working.

4. Diagnosis Aid:

• Biological Staining: Stains cells and tissues to improve visibility under a microscope. Used in histology and cytology.

• Clinical Use: Enables precise diagnosis of illnesses and ailments by taking into account the morphology and structure of cells.

5. Agent Neuroprotective:

• Mechanism: May be helpful in neurodegenerative illnesses by shielding neurons from oxidative damage.

• Clinical Use: Its potential to slow down neurodegeneration and improve cognitive performance is being studied.

Science:

1. Biological Staining:

• Microscopy: This technique is used to dye tissues and cells to improve contrast and visibility under a microscope.

• Research Use: Facilitates comprehensive analysis of cellular architecture and functions in biological research.

2. The Redox Indicator

• Analytical Chemistry: Changes color in response to oxidation state changes, serving as a redox indicator in chemical reactions.

• Research Use: Beneficial for detecting redox reactions in spectrophotometer, titrations, and other analytical procedures.

3. Research on Mitochondria:

• Cellular activity: Effects on cellular respiration and mitochondrial activity were studied.

• Research Use: Researched to comprehend oxidative stress mechanisms and energy metabolism in cellular biology and physiology.

4. Research on Antimicrobials:

• Antimicrobial and Antifungal Properties: Looked at for possible uses in the fight against microbial illnesses.

• Research Use: Developing novel antibacterial methods and assessing efficacy against certain infections.

5. Experimental Physician:

• Adjunct therapy: Investigated for possible use in the treatment of cancer and other disorders where mitochondrial function is involved.

• Research Use: Preclinical and clinical investigations to evaluate the safety and effectiveness of treatments in a range of illness models.

Uses of Methylene Blue in Medicine

Because of its special qualities, methylene blue is a chemical that is highly versatile and has various key medical applications.

1. Methemoglobinemia Treatment:

• State: Hemoglobin loses its capacity to bind and release oxygen efficiently in patients with methemoglobinemia.

• Mechanism: Methylene Blue restores the ability of methemoglobin ($Fe3+$) to carry oxygen by converting it back to functional hemoglobin ($Fe2+$).

• Clinical Use: Treating congenital and acquired methemoglobinemia in an emergency situation to ensure that tissues receive enough oxygen.

2. The remedy for poisoning with cyanide:

• Situation: When cyanide exposure prevents cells from respiring, it results in cyanide poisoning.

• Mechanism: By promoting the transformation of cyanide into less poisonous cyanate, methylene blue helps in detoxification.

• Clinical Use: Applied in conjunction with other medicines to improve cyanide elimination as part of therapy protocols for acute cyanide poisoning.

3. Aid in Diagnosis:

• Biological Staining: Stains cells and tissues to improve visibility under a microscope. Used in histology and cytology.

• Clinical Use: Helps identify aberrant cellular structures and enables precise diagnosis of diseases like bladder cancer.

4. Urinary Antiseptic:

• Situation: Bacterial invasion of the urinary system is the cause of urinary tract infections (UTIs).

• Mechanism: Methylene Blue has antibacterial qualities that combat urinary tract germs.

• Clinical Use: As an adjuvant treatment for UTIs, especially

when the infections are resistant
to traditional antibiotics.

5. Effects of Neuroprotection:

• State: The function of the
neurological system gradually
deteriorates in neurodegenerative
illnesses.

• Mechanism: By defending
neurons against oxidative stress
and promoting mitochondrial
activity, methylene blue may be
able to halt the course of disease.

• Clinical Use: Investigative
treatments to maintain neuronal
integrity and cognitive function
for diseases such as Parkinson's
and Alzheimer's.

6. photodynamics Therapy(PDT):

• Condition: Photodynamic therapy (PDT) uses light-sensitive chemicals to treat a few types of cancer and skin disorders.

• Mechanism: When Methylene Blue is exposed to light, it produces reactive oxygen species, which kill cancer cells on the spot.

• Clinical Use: Shows potential in targeted cancer therapy when used in PDT experimental settings.

7. Supplementary Care in Sepsis:

• State: Sepsis is a potentially fatal illness brought on by the body's reaction to an infection.

• Mechanism: Methylene Blue has the potential to enhance hemodynamic stability and regulate inflammatory responses.

• Clinical Use: Being researched as an adjuvant therapy to improve outcomes and lower fatality rates in sepsis care.

Chapter Seven

Non-Medical of Applications Methylene Blue

Because of its special qualities, Methylene Blue has a wide range of non-medical uses in addition to its medical applications.

1. Biological Staining:

• Microscopy: Staining cells and tissues to improve visibility under a microscope is a common practice in biological and medical laboratories.

• Research: Makes it easier to examine cellular architecture and functions in detail, which is helpful for diagnostics and research.

2. Aquarium Maintenance:

• Fish Health: Used to treat parasite and fungal illnesses in fish, such as fin rot and ich (white spot disease).

• Egg Disinfection: Stops fungi from growing on fish eggs while they are being bred and incubated.

3. Dyeing textiles:

• Historical Use: Although it is less frequent now, methylene blue has been used historically in the textile industry as a dye to color fabrics and fibers.

4. Chemical indicator:

• Analytical Chemistry: Changes color in response to oxidation-reduction states, serving as a redox indicator in chemical reactions.

• Titration: This method improves accuracy in quantitative chemical analysis by identifying the titration's endpoint.

5. Photography:

• Alternative Processes: It serves as a photosensitive dye in alternative photography processes including cyanotype printing.

6. Electron Microscopy:

• Contrast Enhancement: Used in electron microscopy on occasion to enhance contrast and make cellular features more visible.

7. Water Purification:

• Disinfection: Methylene Blue's potential as a disinfectant in water treatment procedures has been investigated in a few applications.

8. Education in Chemistry:

• Demonstrations: Used in educational contexts to illustrate concepts of chemistry, such as color changes and oxidation-reduction reactions.

Safety Observations:

• Although typically safe for the purposes for which they are intended, care should be taken to prevent ingestion or contact with the skin and eyes.

• Adherence to appropriate handling and disposal protocols is crucial in order to mitigate ecological harm and guarantee safety.

Chapter Eight

Taking Safety Measures and Precaution When Using Methylene Blue

When used properly, methylene blue is generally safe, however it's crucial to adhere to safety precautions to reduce hazards and guarantee safe handling:

1. Personal protection Equipment (PPE):

• Gloves and Eye Protection: To avoid skin contact and eye irritation, wear gloves, safety goggles, or a face shield when handling Methylene Blue.

2. Storage and Handling:

• Storage Requirements: To preserve stability, store Methylene Blue in a cool, dry location away from moisture and direct light.

• Sealed Containers: To avoid spillage and contamination, store in tightly sealed containers.

3. How to Prepare and Use It:

• Dilution: Make Methylene Blue solutions as needed, and keep it away from air and light for extended periods of time as this can reduce its potency.

• Accurate Measurement: To guarantee proper dosage and

dilution, use precise measuring equipment.

4. Removal:

• Appropriate Disposal: Get rid of any leftover or out-of-date Methylene Blue in accordance with local laws and hazardous waste disposal requirements.

5. Health Precaution:

Steer clear of extended skin contact. If inadvertent contact occurs, use soap and water to cleanse the affected areas.

• Eye Contact: If Methylene Blue gets into contact with your eyes, rinse them out right away with water for a few minutes.

• Ingestion: Refrain from consuming Methylene Blue. If ingested, get medical help right away and tell them about the product.

6. Particular Points to Remember:

• Allergy Reactions: Keep an eye out for symptoms of allergies, particularly in those who are sensitive, such as skin rashes or breathing difficulties.

• Medical Conditions: People who lack glucose-6-phosphate dehydrogenase (G6PD) should use caution since Methylene Blue can cause hemolysis.

7. Effect on the Environment:

• Environmental Precautions: Use appropriate handling and disposal techniques to reduce pollution and exposure to the environment.

Emergencies Procedures:

• Emergency Contact: In the event of an unintentional exposure or ingestion, keep emergency contact information close at hand.

• Safety Data Sheet (SDS): For comprehensive instructions on handling, storing, and emergency protocols, consult the Safety Data Sheet.

Chapter Nine

DIY Preparation and Dosing at Home

To ensure safety and efficacy, Methylene Blue dosing and preparation for do-it-yourself projects should be done carefully and precisely. Here are some general pointers for dosing and preparing at home:

Sourcing Methylene Blue

It's important to take extra caution when sourcing Methylene Blue for non-medical or do-it-yourself projects to make sure you get a high-quality item fit for its intended usage. The following are broad recommendations for locating Methylene Blue:

1. Identify Reliable Vendors:

• Chemical Suppliers: Seek out trustworthy companies that specialize in providing chemicals and reagents for laboratory use.

• Aquarium Suppliers: Methylene Blue for fish care may be available at certain specialty aquarium stores.

• Online retailers: Methylene Blue is frequently sold on websites that specialize in chemical supplies, such as Amazon, eBay, and similar platforms.

2. Purity and Quality:

• Purity Grade: Verify that the Methylene Blue is pure enough for the use for which it is intended. Technical or analytical grade purity is enough for the majority of non-medical applications.

• Product Specifications: Verify purity and handling instructions by consulting the supplier's Safety Data Sheets (SDS) and product specifications.

3. How to package and handle:

• Packaging: To avoid damage during shipping and storage,

select products that are packaged securely.

• Storage Recommendations: To ensure product integrity, confirm the supplier's suggested storage conditions (e.g., cold, dry place away from light).

4. Client Testimonials and Input:

• Do your research: To determine the dependability and caliber of a supplier's items, look through client testimonials and reviews on their website or on other platforms.

• Advice: Consult forums or reliable sources for advice

relevant to your particular use case (e.g., aquarium maintenance, instructional objectives).

5. Legal Aspects to Take into Account:

• Regulations: Make sure that all local laws and regulations pertaining to the usage, storage, and acquisition of chemicals such as Methylene Blue are followed.

• Permits: To buy and handle specific amounts of Methylene Blue, you might require licenses or permits, depending on your area and planned use.

6. Delivery and Handling Charges:

• Delivery Options: Pick a delivery method based on your requirements for safety, speed, and tracking.

• Handling Fees: When buying chemical materials, be mindful of any additional handling costs or specifications that might be necessary.

Safety Measures:

• **Personal Protective Equipment (PPE):** To avoid skin contact and eye irritation, always wear the proper PPE, such as gloves and eye protection, when handling Methylene Blue.

• **Storage:** To preserve Methylene Blue's stability and efficacy, store it safely and in accordance with supplier guidelines.

• **Disposal:** Follow your local community's hazardous waste disposal requirements for getting rid of any leftover or expired Methylene Blue.

You can efficiently get Methylene Blue for non-medical or do-it-yourself applications while putting safety, quality, and legal compliance first by according to these principles. If you're unsure, speaking with chemical suppliers or subject-matter specialists can offer more advice catered to your particular need.

Preparation Technique

Several methods must be used to prepare Methylene Blue solution, depending on the intended use and concentration. Here are a few typical general preparation methods that are employed:

1. Making a Dilute Solution:

Material Required:

- Methylene Blue Powder

- Distilled Water

- A measuring scale or spoon

• Sterile Container (plastic or glass)

• A magnetic stirrer or stirring stick

Steps:

1. Calculate Concentration:

• Based on your particular application, ascertain the appropriate concentration of the Methylene Blue solution (e.g., aquarium treatment, staining).

2. Measure Methylene Blue:

The right amount of Methylene Blue powder should be measured with a scale or measuring spoon. The amount will vary based on the solution's intended final volume and concentration.

3. Get the Dilute Solution Ready:

• Transfer the measured powdered Methylene Blue to a sterile container.

• To dissolve the powder, add a tiny bit of distilled water. To aid in dissolution, start with a little volume.

4. Mix and Dissolve:

• To promote dissolution, gently swirl the mixture using a magnetic stirrer or stirring rod. Try not to mix too much at once to avoid too much foaming.

5. Progressive Dilution:

• Add additional distilled water gradually while stirring to ensure that all of the Methylene Blue powder has dissolved and the mixture is homogenous.

6. Final Volume Modification:

• To get the appropriate concentration, adjust the solution's final volume by adding extra distilled water as needed. Stir continuously to guarantee consistency.

7. Labeling and Storage:

• Keep the prepared Methylene Blue solution out of direct

sunlight and heat by sealing it tightly.

• Write the concentration, the date of preparation, and any pertinent safety information on the container's label.

2. Preparing the Stock Solution:

Material Required:

• Powdered Methylene Blue

• Distilled Water

• Gradient cylinder or measuring flask

• Sterile Container (plastic or glass)

• Optional magnetic stirrer

Steps:

1. Measure Methylene Blue:

• Measure a greater quantity of Methylene Blue powder appropriate for making a stock solution using an exact measurement device.

2. Get the stock solution ready.

• Transfer the measured Methylene Blue powder straight into a measuring flask or into a sterile, clean container.

3. Add Distilled Water:

• Fill the flask or container with a predetermined amount of distilled water to make up the Methylene

Blue powder. The desired concentration for the stock solution will determine the volume.

4. Mix and Dissolve:

• Using a magnetic stirrer or gently whirling, thoroughly mix the mixture until all of the Methylene Blue powder has dissolved.

5. Dilution for Application:

• Add the required amount of distilled water to the stock solution to dilute it to the desired concentration when it's time to use it. To achieve even dispersion, thoroughly mix.

6. Labeling and Storage:

• Keep the stock solution at the prescribed temperature in a firmly sealed container that is shielded from light.

• Clearly mark the container with the stock solution's concentration, the preparation date, and any handling guidelines.

Safety Observations:

• **Personal Protective Equipment (PPE):** To avoid skin contact and ocular irritation, wear gloves and protective eyewear whenever handling Methylene Blue powder and solutions.

• **Storage:** To preserve stability and efficacy, keep Methylene Blue solutions out of direct sunlight and in a cold, dry location.

• **Disposal:** Get rid of any leftover or expired solutions in accordance with local laws governing the disposal of hazardous waste.

These methods of preparation guarantee that Methylene Blue solutions are made, metered, and handled safely and correctly for a variety of activities, ranging from staining and aquarium maintenance to laboratory research and non-medical purposes. Adapt the methods according to the precise volume and concentration requirements for the desired application.

Dosage Guidelines

Whether Methylene Blue is being used for a medicinal or non-medical purpose, different applications have different dosage recommendations. An outline of dosage considerations for various usage is provided below:

Medical Applications:

1. Methemoglobinemia:

• Adults: Usually given intravenously at a maximum dose of 7 mg/kg, or 1-2 mg/kg of body weight.

• Children: Doses are usually given at lower concentrations and under medical supervision; they can vary depending on age and weight.

2. Poisoning with Cyanide:

• Adults: Intravenous administration at a dose of 1-2 mg/kg body weight.

• Children: Lower dosages given under medical supervision, based on weight.

Non-Medical Applications:

1. Treatment in an aquarium:

• Dosage: Typically, aquarium water contains 0.05 to 0.1 mg/L (milligrams per liter).

• Use: For fungal or parasite illnesses, apply topically as a bath treatment or straight into aquarium water as needed.

2. Natural Staining:

• Concentration: Diluted to different concentrations according to necessary staining intensity and particular staining procedures.

• Use: Improves the visibility of cellular features under microscopy in cytology and histology.

3. Chemical Signal:

• Titration: Add small amounts of an indicator to titration reactions to detect changes in color at the endpoint. This method is mostly used in analytical chemistry.

General Consideration:

• **Accuracy:** To guarantee proper dosing, particularly for medical purposes, use precise measuring instruments (such as calibrated droppers or syringes).

• **Consultation:** Dosing for medicinal purposes should always be decided upon and overseen by medical professionals, taking into account specific patient circumstances.

• **Safety:** Observe handling instructions and safety

precautions to avoid inadvertent exposure or ingestion, especially when handling concentrated solutions.

Chapter Ten

Safety Measures:

• **Personal Protective Equipment (PPE):** To prevent skin contact and eye irritation, wear gloves and protective eyewear when handling Methylene Blue solutions.

• **Storage:** As advised by the supplier, keep Methylene Blue solutions in tightly sealed containers away from light and moisture.

• **Disposal:** Follow local hazardous waste disposal laws when getting rid of leftover or expired Methylene Blue solutions.

The recommended dosage for Methylene Blue varies significantly according on the intended usage, ranging from non-medical uses such as aquarium maintenance to staining in laboratory settings and medicinal treatments. It is important to adhere to the precise dosage guidelines furnished by manufacturers or healthcare experts to guarantee a secure and efficient utilization for your particular purpose.

Practical Use and Applications

Because of its many uses, methylene blue is used in biology, chemistry, medicine, and other fields in practical applications. The following are some real-world applications and uses for Methylene Blue:

Applications in Medicine:

1. Methemoglobinemia Treatment:

• Mechanism: Restores the blood's ability to carry oxygen by converting methemoglobin to hemoglobin.

• Use: As an urgent treatment for methemoglobinemia brought on by drugs, toxins, or genetics.

2. The remedy cyanide poisoning:

• Mechanism: By changing cyanide into less poisonous forms, it aids in the detoxification process.

• Usage: A component of acute cyanide poisoning therapy regimens, particularly for victims of smoke inhalation.

3. Aid in Diagnosis:

• Biological Staining: Stains tissues and cells for microscopic inspection in cytology and histology.

• Use: Improves cell structure contrast and visualization, which helps in disease diagnosis.

4. Urinary Antiseptic:

• Mechanism: Demonstrates antibacterial characteristics against urinary tract bacteria.

• Usage: Adjunct treatment for UTIs, especially when the infection is resistant to traditional antibiotics.

5. Effects of Neuroprotection:

• Mechanism: Promotes mitochondrial health and shields neurons from oxidative damage.

• Use: Being researched for possible therapeutic advantages

in neurodegenerative illnesses such as Parkinson's and Alzheimer's.

Non medical Application:

6. Aquarium Maintenance:

● **Use:** Add at prescribed amounts to aquarium water to treat fish diseases caused by fungi and parasites.

7. Using Biological Staining in Studies

● **Use:** Improves cellular structure visibility under microscopy, which is important for biological and medical research.

8. Chemical Signal:

● **Use:** In analytical chemistry, it serves as a redox indicator to identify endpoint color changes in titrations and chemical reactions.

9. Photography:

● Use: Because of its light-sensitive characteristics, it is utilized in alternative photographic processes like cyanotype printing.

10. Textiles Dyeing:

● **Use:** Although less frequently used in contemporary applications, historically used as a dye for fabrics and textiles.

Applications in Research and Education:

• **Research on mitochondria:** Examines how these structures affect both healthy and unhealthy conditions with regard to cellular respiration and mitochondrial function.

• **Chemical Education:** In educational settings, demonstrates the fundamentals of color changes and oxidation-reduction reactions.

• **Electron Microscopy:** Improves contrast to make cellular structures easier to see in electron microscopy.

Safety Observations:

• **Handling:** When handling concentrated solutions, wear the proper personal protective equipment (PPE), such as gloves and eye protection.

• **Storage:** To ensure stability, keep Methylene Blue stored in tightly sealed containers away from light and moisture.

• **Disposal:** Get rid of leftover or outdated solutions in accordance with regional laws governing dangerous substances.

The numerous uses of Methylene Blue highlight its value in scientific research, medical treatments, and other practical applications, as well as its adaptability and advantageous qualities in a variety of fields.

Common Issues

The following are some typical problems that arise when Methylene Blue is used in different applications:

Medical Issues:

1. Hemolysis in G6PD Deficiency:

• **Issue:** Methylene Blue can trigger hemolysis (destruction of red blood cells) in individuals with glucose-6-phosphate dehydrogenase (G6PD) deficiency.

• **Precaution:** Avoid use or use with extreme caution under medical supervision in patients with known or suspected G6PD deficiency.

2. Overdose and Toxicity:

• **Issue:** Excessive doses of Methylene Blue can lead to toxicity symptoms, including methemoglobinemia (blue discoloration of skin), respiratory distress, and potential organ damage.

• **Precaution:** Strictly adhere to recommended dosing guidelines and monitor patients closely during administration.

3. Interaction with Medications:

• **Issue:** Methylene Blue can interact with various medications, including serotonergic agents, leading to serotonin syndrome.

• **Precaution:** Assess medication history and potential interactions before administering Methylene Blue, particularly in patients taking antidepressants or other serotonergic drugs.

Non-Medical Issues:

4. Staining and Discoloration:

- **Issue:** Methylene Blue can stain skin, clothing, and other surfaces due to its intense blue color.

- **Precaution:** Use appropriate PPE during handling to avoid skin contact. Clean spills immediately with appropriate solvents.

5. Effect on the Environment:

- **Issue:** Improper disposal of Methylene Blue can lead to environmental contamination and harm aquatic ecosystems.

- **Precaution:** Dispose of Methylene Blue solutions according to local regulations for hazardous chemicals. Consider eco-friendly alternatives or treatment methods where possible.

6. Storage and Stability:

• **Issue:** Improper storage conditions (e.g., exposure to light, moisture) can degrade Methylene Blue, reducing its effectiveness.

• **Precaution:** Store Methylene Blue in tightly sealed, light-resistant containers in a cool, dry place. Follow supplier recommendations for storage and shelf-life.

7. Safety during Handling:

• **Issue:** Handling concentrated solutions of Methylene Blue without proper PPE can lead to skin irritation and eye damage.

• **Precaution:** Always wear gloves, safety goggles, and protective clothing when handling Methylene Blue solutions. Avoid inhalation and ingestion.

Research and Educational Issues:

8. Quality and Consistency:

• **Issue:** Variations in purity and quality of Methylene Blue can affect experimental results and staining outcomes.

• **Precaution:** Source Methylene Blue from reputable suppliers and verify purity and specifications before use in research or educational settings.

9. Application Specificity:

• **Issue:** Different applications (e.g., biological staining, chemical indicator) may require specific concentrations and preparation techniques for optimal results.

• **Precaution:** Follow established protocols and guidelines for each application to achieve desired outcomes and avoid unnecessary complications.

Addressing these common issues with careful consideration and adherence to safety protocols ensures the effective and responsible use of Methylene Blue across medical, scientific, and practical applications.